COUNSEL FOR THE CARETAKER

"A navigation guide for skilled nursing care"

Faith A. Turner

Counsel for The Caretaker

A Navigation Guide for Skilled Nursing Care

Copyright © 2017

Tampa, FL

Published 2017 by Faith A. Turner

All rights reserved. No portion of this book may be reproduced, photocopied, stored, or transmitted in any form-except by prior approval of publisher.

Cover design:

Book Layout Assisted: www.diverseskillcenter.com

Printed in the United States of America

ISBN-13:978-1975632854

ISBN-10:1975632850

Table of Contents

Acknowledgements 4

Introduction 5

Chapter 1 – Hospitalization 7

Chapter 2 – Finding A Facility 11

Chapter 3 – Found A Facility, Now What? 15

Chapter 4 – Insurance & Long-Term Care 21

Chapter 5 – Encouragement for the Care-Taker 29

Contacts 32

Dedication

This book is dedicated to my loving parents

Judith and Willie Nelson.

You aren't here alive to see this accomplishment but, I know you are still watching over me. I'm so grateful to God for giving me you as parents. Before you left this earth, you poured out and instilled in me all that I have become and will become. You were my biggest cheerleaders. You saw me through some rough times in my life. You were my strength. Most of all, I am so appreciative you introduced me to Christ, the Lover of my soul!

I love and miss you both greatly!

Acknowledgements

I would like to acknowledge the Holy Spirit for the revelation of this book and Cynthia Johnson for helping me birth it out. I appreciate you greatly!

Introduction

Hello,

My name is Faith. If you have this book, I'm sure you are looking for help regarding the process of care after hospitalization. I have over 16 years of experience in the healthcare field. Over the years, I have learned the processes and have encountered so many caretakers not having all the answers they need. The social workers at the hospitals do not have all the answers, and let's be honest; most aren't willing to help you find the answers. You are left pretty much to figure it all out. Well, look no further. This guide will give you all the answers you need step by step. You will find this very informative and easy to follow without you becoming more frustrated or stressed. As I tell many, NEVER FEAR, FAITH IS HERE! Let's begin...

Faith A. Turner

Chapter One

"Hospitalization"

Suddenly, you as the caretaker find yourself in the hospital with a loved one, and the diagnosis given requires another level of care to rehabilitate before transitioning home, such as dementia, that is progressively getting worse will require long-term care. At this point, you are somewhat stressed and feeling a little bit overwhelmed. You have never been in this position before. Take a breath! Take another! And another! You are going to get through this successfully! It's important that you begin to take one step at a time. The social worker at the hospital will start a discharge plan. The plan will include a date given to discharge the patient from the hospital with instructions. Typically, they ask the family to tour different facilities. You want to make sure the facility accepts your insurance. Most families prefer to choose one within 10 miles of their homes to be able to visit more often. The social worker will send out a referral, which is the basic information about your loved one, to different facilities to give you options to choose from. The acceptance from the facility of your loved one will be based on your insurance and the ability of the facility to meet the needs of the patient. FYI: Do not allow them to push your relative into any facility just to get them out of theirs. You need to know your rights. You have the right to appeal the discharge, which they will not make known to you. If you feel your loved one isn't ready medically for the next level of care then you should exercise this right. If you feel he or she is ready, then it is time for the next step. Choose a facility that will not only meet the needs of your loved one but also will exceed them.

Notes

Notes

Chapter Two
"Finding a Facility"

First things first. You want to do your homework first prior to touring the facility that interests you. You need to view the medicare.gov website to give you the latest rating of the facility as well as its last state inspection. Call the facility to verify if they accept your insurance, what services they provide and whether you can stop by for a tour. When touring the site, I recommend that it be done after hours during the week or on the weekend. This will give you great insight into how the facility runs after administration leaves. Pay attention to staffing, cleanliness, and assess any residents you may see. Ask them questions about the staff and do they like the facility. Take notice of their appearance; are they groomed, are their clothes clean, do they appear happy? If you tour doing the day with the facility personnel make sure you have a list of questions to ask prior to touring. Ask questions like, do you have RN's on staff 24 hours a day, what is the staffing ratio, are activities available, what are the visiting hours, what specialty services are offered, and how often is therapy done? If your loved one needs long-term care, make sure you mention this up front. For those with Medicare, which is the most lucrative insurance, please be aware of facilities using all their allotted days then forcing your loved ones out into other facility, possibly of a lower quality, and further away from their families. This can cause lots of strain. Please remember do not decide right away. Take your time to make the right decision for you and your loved one.

Notes

Notes

Chapter Three
"You Found a Facility, NOW WHAT?"

Finally, you have chosen a facility that best suits your family's needs. While there, take note of all the administration names and phone numbers. The administrator and social workers are your go-to people to get your concerns resolved immediately. Facilities want grievances and complaints down to a bare minimum. Remember you are a PRIORITY! LET YOUR VOICE BE HEARD! You are your loved one's advocate. Get to know the list of resident rights given to every person admitted to the facility. If you don't know the power you have, you will never use it. Nursing and other clinical staff are required by law to give updated information on every shift showing sometimes, in detail, the progress of the patients. The patient and you are the POA can have full access to such information.

You might ask, "What does POA mean?" It means POWER OF ATTORNEY. Basically, it is when someone is no longer able to handle their financial and health care affairs they give someone they trust power of attorney to handle these affairs on their behalf.

Advance Care Directives are very important to have. These are things such as living wills, POA, and DNR, also known as Do Not Resuscitate. The social worker at the facility will help explain in full details of each of them are and how to obtain them. I recommend you visit in the later hours and do pop ups to make sure your loved one is being cared for attentively. Ask about staffing hours, they should be somewhere in the facility easy for you to see. Make sure the call light is in place and it is being answered appropriately. If you have concerns, please follow up with the proper personnel to get it resolved. Speak with the therapy department to get updates regarding the status of your loved one's ability to go home, and function as independently as possible. The social worker will be the individual to help assist you with discharge planning to go home with minimal concerns. He or she can make sure there is a bed, oxygen, IV, and wound care all set up prior to discharge. The goal is to ultimately prevent the patient from coming back to the hospital. Your insurance typically covers such benefit.

Notes

Chapter Four

"Everything You Need to Know about Insurance including Long Term Care"

Medicare is the best insurance for a skilled nursing setting, but will not provide you with the coverage needed for long-term care. Medicare covers 100 days. Days 1-20 are covered @ 100%. Days 21-100, there is a co-pay of 164.40 per day through the 100th day. If you don't have a secondary insurance plan such as Blue Cross Blue Shield to cover, you must pay privately out of pocket. It is important that you discuss with the business office manager a payment plan or start the Medicaid process, also known as ICP Medicaid, as soon as possible. HMO's such as Humana, Care-plus, and United functions as Medicare replacement plans. You will need a secondary payor for these insurances as well. You need to know that these insurances will not continue to authorize coverage if your loved one isn't progressing in therapy or if they came only for IV therapy and it to be discontinue. They will stop payment immediately and will no longer pay for the rest of the stay. You can always dis-enroll from such plans and will become a Medicare primary patient the beginning of the following month. This will allow for more therapy however; you will still need to pay a copayment.

There are certain requirements needed for ICP Medicaid. You can't have over $2,000 in the bank or assets that amount to such. You can have a house, and a car. Your 401k plan or a life insurance policy can't exceed $2,000. If you are over these assets the facility will not be able to assist in the application. You will need to find an elder law attorney; most facilities have at least one contact. For the spouse that may be applying for their loved one, make sure to submit your bills to show you depend on the income. The facility doesn't have a decision on how much your portion will be; the state makes such decisions. Typically, most of the income will go to the facility except for 105 dollars. The money can be allocated for whatever you want. Most facilities have residents trust accounts that the money can be deposited into, which you can have complete control over. If you are a family member obtaining funds from the account, make sure you return all receipts or items purchased from the facility so they can keep track of the account so you can be in right standing with the state if they ever get audited. The following is a list of specific documents needed for the Medicaid application. Gather all that applies to you. If you don't reveal everything and the state recovers it, the application will possibly be denied. You will want to be as truthful as possible.

Personal Information

- Driver License
- Birth Certificate
- Passport
- Alien Registration
- Military Identification
- Social Security Card
- Medicare Card or HMO card

Household Information

- Verification of Residency (rent receipt)
- Utility bills (lights, water, electric, etc.)

Verification of Income

- SSI Benefits (proof of gross amount)
- Verification of Pension Benefits (including any deductions)
- Verification of Other Retirement Benefits

- Verification of VA Benefits
- Verification of Income from Property
- Verification of Income from Investments or any Interest-Bearing Account
- Verification of Bank Statements (all accounts)

Assets

- Verification and Proof of Automobiles
- Life Insurance Policy and Cash Value
- Any Real Property Other Than Homestead
- Any Stocks, Bonds, IRA
- Any Prepaid Burial

Notes

Notes

Notes

Chapter Five

"Encouragement for the Caretaker"

Along this journey of being a care taker you must make sure you take time out for yourself. You can't keep putting everyone before yourself or you will become ill and no longer will be any good to anyone else. Know that your labor of love isn't in vain. May you be strengthened and have peace that surpasses all understanding. May you receive help from many of your family members so you can rest and be restored. You are valuable! Don't become weary and keep doing well!

Notes

Contact Us

For any comments, bookings, bulk information, or free consultations, please contact me at:

Faith Turner

kingdomextension@gmail.com

(813)586-3550

Information in Chapter 4 is referenced to

https://www.dcf.state.fl.us/programs/access/docs/icp_brochure.pdf

www.ingramcontent.com/pod-product-compliance
Lightning Source LLC
Chambersburg PA
CBHW050035230526
45470CB00003B/1287